Sacroiliac Pain
UNDERSTANDING THE PELVIC GIRDLE MUSCULOSKELETAL METHOD℠

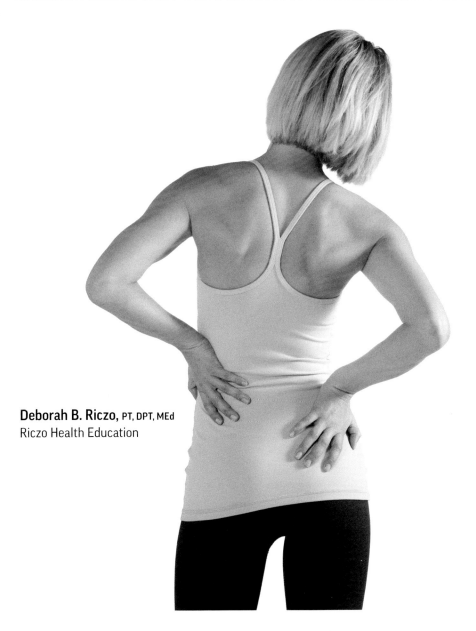

Deborah B. Riczo, PT, DPT, MEd
Riczo Health Education

© 2018 Deborah B. Riczo, PT, DPT, MEd

All rights reserved. No part of this publication may be reproduced, stored in a retrieval system or transmitted in any form or by any means that includes but is not limited to electronic, mechanical, photocopying or recording with the exception of brief quotations embodied in critical articles and reviews.

The procedures and practices described in this book should be implemented in a manner consistent with professional standards set for the circumstances that apply in each situation. Every effort has been made to confirm accuracy of the information presented and to correctly relate generally accepted practices.

The author, editor and publisher cannot accept responsibility for errors or exclusions or for the outcome of the application of the material presented herein. There is no expressed or implied warranty of this book or information imparted by it.

Designed, copyedited and published by OPTP.
3800 Annapolis Lane N, Suite 165, Minneapolis, MN 55447
OPTP.com

ISBN #978-1-942798-13-2

Illegal to reproduce

Contents

Section One

    Awareness by understanding

        Do I have sacroiliac dysfunction?..1
- Where is the pain?
- What kind of pain is it?
- Why would I have it?

        What is sacroiliac dysfunction?..2-7
- The anatomy of the sacroiliac joint
- The role of the muscles
- Problems with movement and pain
- Sleep
- Command central, the brain

        Taking the next step..8

        References...9

Section Two

    The Pelvic Girdle Musculoskeletal Method℠ (PGM Method℠)

        Step 1. Determining which exercises are best for you 10-19
- Breathing
- Pelvic balancing exercises

        Step 2. Activating your deep core muscles 20-22
- Activating your deep core, exercise #4

        Step 3. Stretching your buttocks, hips and low back;
        achieving balance between the sides of your body 23-30

        Step 4. Begin a walking program... 31

        Step 5. Progress to other physical activities that you enjoy, make healthy choices 32

        References..33

Section Three

    Other helpful information

        Using a sacroiliac belt 34

        FAQs..35-37

        Exercise planner 38

        Stretching planner..39

        Goals..40

Introduction

Sacroiliac dysfunction affects an estimated 10-30 percent of persons with non-specific low back pain and is often present with complaints of hip and leg pain on the same side.[1,2] It often goes undiagnosed and may actually be one of the sources of low back pain.

The Pelvic Girdle Musculoskeletal Method[SM] is a program that allows the individual to monitor his or her own signs and symptoms and approach them in a logical, sequential fashion using sound exercises. These exercises are designed to address muscle imbalances, weakness, and strength. This program is holistic in its approach and educates the individual regarding the important role relaxation, stress management, and mindfulness play in managing pain. This program is NOT about manipulating the sacroiliac joint.

I have three purposes in writing this book:

1. To provide basic education, screening guidelines, and exercises to the person affected with symptoms of sacroiliac dysfunction.

2. To empower a person to take control of his or her health, be mindful, choose wellness, and, in doing so, gradually improve their day-to-day functioning and overall quality of life.

3. To provide an easy education tool that can supplement a healthcare provider's education and treatment of sacroiliac dysfunction in an efficient manner.

I dedicate this handbook to my first grandchild, Annabelle Jane. You light up my life and everyone you meet. May you forever keep your love and spontaneity of life! In addition, I would like to thank my husband John for his love and understanding of the many hours I have spent at the computer literally throughout my career; my daughter Alexa Lee for her love and continual support, and for being the model in this book; my son Christopher for always challenging me; and my dear friend and colleague, Mary Morrison, PT, DScPT, MHS, GCS, for her encouragement and thoughtful review of this book. I would also like to thank all the patients that have crossed my path. I have learned something from each and every one of you.

SECTION ONE

Awareness by understanding

Do I have sacroiliac dysfunction?

Where is the pain?
Place your hand in the small of your back on one side and then slide it down your back until it is below your waist. This is the area where pain usually starts (Figure 1). It can stay in this area or fluctuate side to side, and can be present with low back, hip, buttock, groin, thigh and calf pain.

What kind of pain is it?
Pain can range from very sharp to dull and aching and usually increases with movement such as getting out of a chair or car, stair climbing, walking and running. Pain can also be increased by lying flat or driving. Sometimes it will vary from day to day and week to week, having highs and lows and it can even change sides of the body.

Why would I have it?
It is most common during pregnancy and after the baby is born and may last for years for some women.[3,4]

Men can have sacroiliac dysfunction, too. It can occur in someone who has had a lumbar fusion or multiple abdominal or pelvic surgeries.[5] Experiencing a fall (especially on your buttock) or motor vehicle accident might also result in the onset of sacroiliac pain.

Both young and old can be affected. A young person may experience pain from a sport or activity. It can also happen when someone who is not physically fit tries a new activity that may be too advanced for them, or by jumping down hard and landing on one leg.

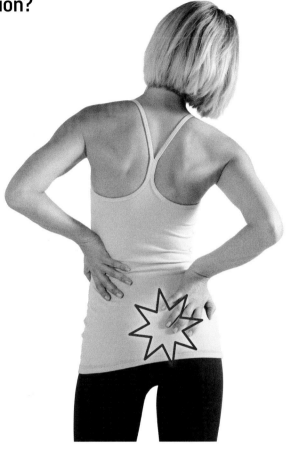

Figure 1. Right-sided pain example.

Problems on one side of the body that affect the way a person walks—like arthritis, torn ligaments, scoliosis, or anything involving the hip, knee or ankle—can contribute to sacroiliac dysfunction, as the muscles may be overworking on one side. This is why people should consider assistive devices that help them walk more normally and consult a physical therapist if they are having difficulty walking.

What is sacroiliac dysfunction?

The anatomy of the sacroiliac joint

The sacroiliac joint is between the sacrum and hip bones (Figure 2).

The pelvis is made up of your sacrum, your coccyx (tailbone), and hip bones or ilium (right and left sides).

The sacroiliac joint is an important shock absorber for your body.

The joint is held together by ligaments and muscles that also affect your hip and low back movements (Figures 3 and 4). Ligaments are important because they hold bones together while allowing some motion between the bones. How much motion the ligaments allow varies from joint to joint.

Research has shown that there is very little movement possible at this joint due to the design of the joint as well as numerous and strong ligaments, and this motion decreases with age.[6,7]

Like other joints, the sacroiliac joint can become inflamed and painful, which can be due to various forms of arthritis, such as gout, rheumatoid arthritis, psoriasis and ankylosing spondylitis. This can stem from a trauma (fall, car accident, etc.) or from wear and tear on the back and pelvic area. Other risk factors for developing arthritic changes in the spine and sacrum are repetitive and awkward postures, heavy workloads, being overweight, being deconditioned, abdominal surgeries (weak core muscles) and genetics.

These painful symptoms may initiate in the joint, but they can involve surrounding tissues and even radiate into the pelvis, groin, buttock and down the leg.[8]

However, some people with sacroiliac pain symptoms do not have inflammation in the actual sacroiliac joint, but in tissues outside of the joint (ligaments, fascia, nerves and muscles). Physicians may use imaging techniques or an injection in the sacroiliac joint to confirm whether the joint is inflamed.

Whether the pain is in the joint or from tissues outside the joint, the conservative approach to treatment involves physician-guided medication (including anti-inflammatories) and what we will be discussing in this book: a holistic approach to health and wellness that includes targeted exercises.

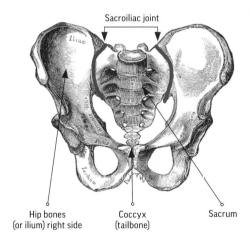

Figure 2. Pelvis[a]

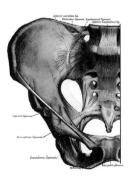

Figure 3. Ligaments at the front of the pelvis[b]

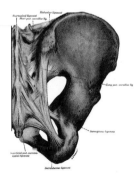

Figure 4. Ligaments at the back of the pelvis[c]

The role of the muscles

If muscles are too tight or overstretched (weak) or have been injured, there can often be an imbalance that produces uneven forces on the joints, causing extra wear and tear. This results in inflammation and pain.[9] You can think of this like a tent that is held too tightly on one side by the tie-down stakes (Figure 5). Tight muscles and inflammation can cause pressure on nerves in the pelvic girdle and can cause pain that travels into the pelvis, buttocks, groin, thigh or calf.[10]

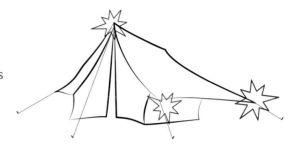

Figure 5. Tent tied down too tightly on one side

We have layers of muscle, from deep to superficial that work in a coordinated way in order for us to function well.

The deep hip rotator muscles (Figure 6) can often tighten up on one side of the buttock and make it difficult to move normally. This can happen when there is weakness in the superficial muscles, specifically the gluteus maximus and gluteus medius.

The deep hip rotator muscles (most well known is the piriformis muscle) attach to the femur or leg bone (Figure 6).

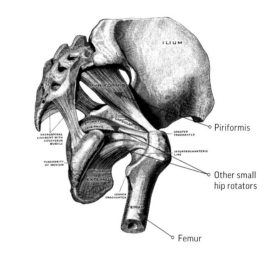

Figure 6. Deep hip rotators

The superficial muscles in the hip area are cut away in this diagram (Figure 7), showing the same small, deep muscles that attach to the femur or leg bone. This is why good rehabilitation exercises involve regaining a balance in all the muscles in the hips, low back, and trunk. They all work together. Many exercises people typically do work to strengthen the superficial muscles. We need to work on both.

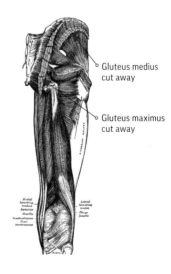

Figure 7. Deep hip rotators[d,e]

The diaphragm muscle sits under our rib cage and is part of the deep muscle system (Figure 8). It is the muscle most responsible for breathing. The back portion of this muscle actually attaches to the middle and lower back vertebrae. When the diaphragm functions normally, there is rhythmical movement in the rib cage, upper and lower vertebrae (small bones of the spine), and intestines. This is important in normal blood flow to these areas and helps maintain a healthy gut. This is why breath awareness and good breathing in general is an important part of this exercise program.

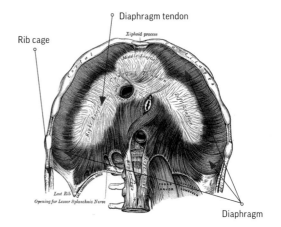

Figure 8. Diaphragm[f]

The pelvic floor muscles are also part of the deep muscle system in the pelvic girdle (Figure 9). They can be tight and painful or weak and cause problems with leaking urine, incontinence, or painful intercourse. Urinary incontinence is a common problem in persons with low back pain.[11]

Following the program in this book will often improve these symptoms. A women's health physical therapist is specially trained in pelvic floor issues and can be of great assistance in addressing these problems.

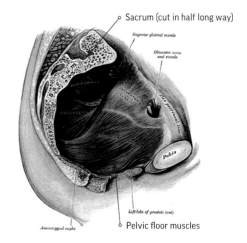

Figure 9. Pelvic Floor Muscles[g]

The transversus abdominus is the deepest layer of the abdominals and is also part of the deep muscle system (Figure 10). When it is weak a person presents with a belly or "pouch." This is another muscle that is often neglected with many exercise programs. This muscle directly wraps around the waist to the lower back muscles/fascia. It is important for good functioning of the trunk and pelvic girdle, which includes the sacroiliac joint.[9]

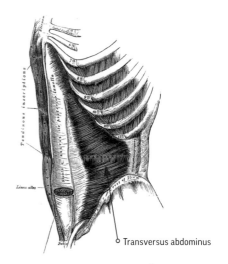

Figure 10. Deep abdominals[h]

The multifidus is the deepest spinal muscle and coordinates with other deep muscles (diaphragm, pelvic floor, transversus abdominus) in normal functioning.[9] When this muscle is weak the more superficial back muscles, including the erector spinae, need to work harder, which can cause them to tighten up, making it difficult to move normally and contribute to back and sacroiliac pain (Figures 11 and 12).

The superficial abdominal muscles are movers of our trunk (Figure 13). They help with support of our spine from the front of the body and are often weak. When these superficial muscles are weak we have increased stresses on our spine and pelvis.

As you can see, our bodies are like a fine orchestra, complex and amazing. The exercises in the next section (Section Two: The Pelvic Girdle Musculoskeletal Method℠) are designed to balance the muscles in your pelvis, strengthen and coordinate your deep core muscles, and balance tightness between the sides of your body. This will get the sound of your orchestra back on track!

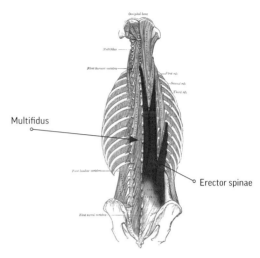

Figure 11. Multifidus (deep) and Erector Spinae (superficial)

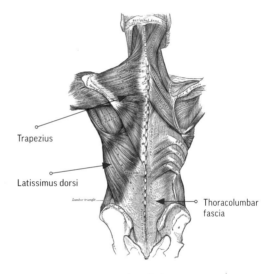

Figure 12. Superficial muscles/fascia of the back[i]

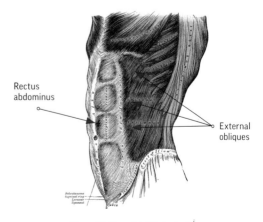

Figure 13. Superficial Abdominals[j]

Sacroiliac Pain, Understanding the Pelvic Girdle Musculoskeletal Method℠ | 5

Problems with movement and pain

Pain can be scary and cause us to be fearful of moving. We often associate the pain with damage to our bodies and become afraid of doing more damage. This thinking may cause us not to move normally, affecting our functioning during day-to-day tasks.

After the first three to six weeks of the onset of pain, research has shown that, in most people, pain is not related to damage but rather to inflammation and nerve sensitivity. Once a nerve or other tissues are irritated, they become irritable, meaning that it takes less to cause pain. That is why it is recommended to avoid or modify activities accordingly to allow the tissues to heal. For example, people whose symptoms are irritated with prolonged sitting may modify by using a standing desk for portions of their work day. The areas of our brain that process our original pain actually shift to the "emotional circuitry" area after approximately one year of chronic pain.[12,13]

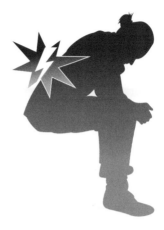

The best thing to remember is pain that has been with you for a while does not necessarily equal damage. Once the initial injury is over, your tissues generally heal.

Fear of moving because you think you will cause more damage, and fear or anxiety regarding your future can make your pain worse. This is due to the hormones that are produced from fear, stress, and anxiety.

In addition, when we become less active we become weaker, in general, having less energy for the things we love to do and only doing what we have to do. This can lead to depression, relationship problems, etc. That is where the deep breathing exercises on page 12 of this book will be very helpful in calming down the nervous system.

The longer we have high anxiety regarding the pain, the more sensitive our brains become to any stimulation; it doesn't even have to be painful stimulation.[14,15] Sometimes just a light touch or wearing certain clothes can feel painful. It is like the floodgates are open to our brain and all stimulation is pouring in.

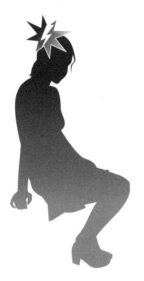

Sleep

These "floodgates" to our brain are even more open at night when we do not have the distractions of our daily life. This can affect getting a good night's rest, which is necessary so our bodies can rejuvenate. These tips may help you get comfortable in bed.

First, make sure your mattress is not contributing to your pain. Your mattress may look fine but if it is 9 or 10 years old it may be time to replace it. Try sleeping on a different mattress (friend's house, hotel, different room in your house), if possible, to compare your sleep.

Second, when sleeping on your side try a pillow between your legs (or even two if it is a thin pillow) with hips and knees comfortably bent and back somewhat straight. You do not want to be in a tightly curled position as that flexed position is harder on your spinal discs. When sleeping on your back a small pillow or roll under your knees may be helpful. It is not advisable to sleep on your stomach due to the pressures on your neck in this position. If, however, that is the most comfortable position for you to fall asleep in, just try to change positions during the night.

Third, diaphragmatic breathing (p. 12) and consciously relaxing and letting go of the day are helpful techniques. There are many relaxation apps available to help you (for example CALM, or Headspace).

A lack of sleep, especially over time, can heighten our perception of pain and the associated anxiety. It can gain momentum on its own like a snowball going down a big hill.

There are therapies available to help with sleep problems. Cognitive behavioral therapy (CBT) can be very helpful. For more tips for improving sleep visit the National Sleep Foundation at thensf.org. Talk to your doctor if you continue to have difficulty sleeping to rule out a sleep disorder and receive guidance.

Command central, the brain

The reason for discussing what we know about how we process pain and other relationships, like sleep, is that we can influence the process. We can stop the snowball before it rolls down the hill, even if it is partway down!

Research has shown that understanding how the brain processes pain and how our behaviors and beliefs about pain affect our brain and nerve sensitivity will dramatically improve our functioning.[12]

Taking the next step

Be open to trusting your body and believe you can improve your functioning.

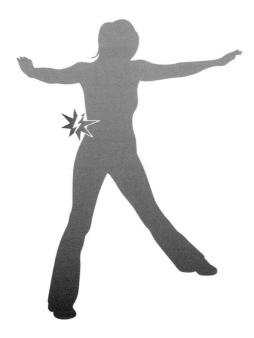

Use the screening tools and exercises in the remainder of this book to address any differences you find between the right and left sides of your body.

As you advance your exercises, look at exercise as a way to become more fit as opposed to getting rid of pain. Looking at exercise through this "lens" will take the focus off pain and instead put it on being the best you inside and out.

Begin a daily walking program or stationary bike program at whatever level you can, along with the exercises in the next section. Regular exercise is a very important part of wellness. Make a decision to increase your activity. Use a calendar to mark each day's session, and note any progress. It will be easier to see how small changes add up over a week or month. If you want to build in a reward system at week's end, go for it. It is not necessary to increase time or speed daily, but hopefully each week you will be able to increase this a little. Faster is not better, at least in the beginning.

Remember to breathe and feel relaxed, not all tensed up, which tightens your muscles. We will talk more about this in the next section. And check with your doctor before beginning a new exercise program!

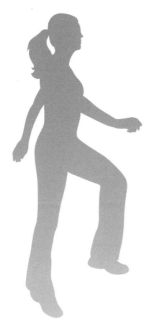
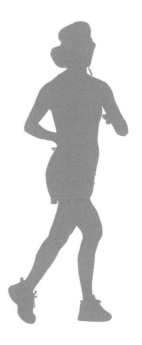

References

1. Bernard TN, Kirkaldy-Willis WH. Recognizing specific characteristics of nonspecific low back pain. *Clin Orthop*. 1987;(217):266-280.

2. Visser LH, Nijssen PG, N, Tijssen CC, van Middendorp JJ, Schieving J. Sciatica-like symptoms and the sacroiliac joint: clinical features and differential diagnosis. *Eur Spine J*. 2013;22(7):1657-1664. doi:http://dx.doi.org/10.1007/s00586-013-2660-5.

3. Katonis P, Kampouroglou A, Aggelopoulos A, et al. Pregnancy-related low back pain. *Hippokratia*. 2011;15(3):205-210.

4. Stuge B. Pelvic girdle pain: examination, treatment, and the development and implementation of the European guidelines | The Chartered Society of Physiotherapy. *ACPWH J*. 2012;111:5-12.

5. DePalma MJ, Ketchum JM, Saullo TR. Etiology of chronic low back pain in patients having undergone lumbar fusion. *Pain Med Malden Mass*. 2011;12(5):732-739. doi:10.1111/j.1526-4637.2011.01098.x.

6. Goode A, Hegedus EJ, Sizer P, Brismee J-M, Linberg A, Cook CE. Three-Dimensional Movements of the Sacroiliac Joint: A Systematic Review of the Literature and Assessment of Clinical Utility. *J Man Manip Ther*. 2008;16(1):25-38. doi:10.1179/106698108790818639.

7. Tullberg T, Blomberg S, Branth B, Johnsson R. Manipulation does not alter the position of the sacroiliac joint. A roentgen stereophotogrammetric analysis. *Man Ther*. 1999;4(1):50. doi:10.1016/S1356-689X(99)80013-7.

8. Matlick D, Dressendorfer R. Sacroiliac Joint Dysfunction. Richman S, ed. *CINAHL Rehabilitation Guide*. September 2017. http://search.ebscohost.com/login.aspx?direct=true&db=rrc&AN=T708569&site=eds-live. Accessed December 7, 2018.

9. Lee, DG. *The Pelvic Girdle: An Integration of Clinical Expertise and Research*. 4th ed. Churchill Livingstone; 2011.

10. Fortin JD, Vilensky JA, Merkel GM. Can the Sacroiliac Joint Cause Sciatica? *Pain Physician*. 2003;(6):269-271.

11. Cassidy T, Fortin A, Kaczmer S, Shumaker JTL, Szeto J, Madill SJ. Relationship Between Back Pain and Urinary Incontinence in the Canadian Population. *Phys Ther*. 2017;97(4):449-454. doi:10.1093/ptj/pzx020.

12. Butler D. *Explain Pain*. 2nd edition. NOI Group; 2013.

13. O'Sullivan P, Caneiro JP, O'Keeffe M, O'Sullivan K. Unraveling the Complexity of Low Back Pain. *J Orthop Sports Phys Ther*. November 2016. doi:10.2519/jospt.2016.0609.

14. Hashmi J, Baliki M, Apkarian V. Shape shifting pain: chronification of back pain shifts brain representation from nociceptive to emotional circuits. *Brain J Neurol*. 2013;136(9):2751-2768. doi:10.1093/brain/awt211.

15. Louw A. *Why Do I Hurt?* 1 edition. S.l.: Orthopedic Physical Therapy Products; 2013.

a. Gray, Henry. "Male pelvis." Bartleby.com, FIG. 241. *Anatomy of the Human Body*, 1918. http://www.bartleby.com/107/illus241.html

b. Gray, Henry. "Articulations of pelvis. Anterior view. (Quain.)" Bartleby.com, FIG. 319. *Anatomy of the Human Body*, 1918. http://www.bartleby.com/107/illus319.html

c. Gray, Henry. "Articulations of pelvis. Posterior view. (Quain.)" Bartleby.com, FIG. 320. *Anatomy of the Human Body*, 1918. http://www.bartleby.com/107/illus320.html

d. Gray, Henry. "Muscles of the gluteal and posterior femoral regions." Bartleby.com, FIG. 434. *Anatomy of the Human Body*, 1918. http://www.bartleby.com/107/illus434.html

e. Gray, Henry. "Muscles of the iliac and anterior femoral regions." Bartleby.com, FIG. 430. *Anatomy of the Human Body*, 1918. http://www.bartleby.com/107/illus430.html

f. Gray, Henry. "The diaphragm. Under surface." Bartleby.com, FIG. 391. *Anatomy of the Human Body*, 1918. http://www.bartleby.com/107/illus391.html

g. Gray, Henry. "Left Levator ani from within." Bartleby.com, FIG. 404. *Anatomy of the Human Body*, 1918. http://www.bartleby.com/107/illus319.html

h. Gray, Henry. "The Transversus abdominis, Rectus abdominis, and Pyramidalis." Bartleby.com, FIG. 397. *Anatomy of the Human Body*, 1918. http://www.bartleby.com/107/illus397.html

i. Gray, Henry. "Muscles connecting the upper extremity to the vertebral column." Bartleby.com, FIG. 409. *Anatomy of the Human Body*, 1918. http://www.bartleby.com/107/illus409.html

j. Gray, Henry. "The Obliquus externus abdominis." Bartleby.com, FIG. 392. *Anatomy of the Human Body*, 1918. http://www.bartleby.com/107/illus392.html

SECTION TWO

The Pelvic Girdle Musculoskeletal Method℠ (PGM Method℠)

What is the PGM Method?

This method is a combination of self-screening tools, simple specific exercises, and education to identify and treat sacroiliac dysfunction. This method was developed by Deborah Riczo, PT, DPT, MEd, and is founded on evidence-based practice and clinical experience of over 30 years.

Step 1. Determining which exercises are best for you

As you go through this section on exercise, use the **Exercise Planner** at the very end of this book (page 38) to help you organize your exercise routine.

Circle which **bones** are tender for you in your pelvis *using the photos on the following page* (Figure 14). These will be your "bony tenderness signs" that will help guide you when you need to do the following exercises.

On the front of your body

- Feel the prominent hip bones below your waist on both sides (this is your ASIS or anterior superior iliac spine). Circle the side that is most tender. If both are equally tender, circle both sides.

- Feel the pubic bones on each side in the low center of your trunk. Circle the side that is most tender. If equally tender circle both sides.

On the back of your body

- Feel the bony small prominence below your waist on each side of your sacrum (this is your PSIS or posterior superior iliac spine). If you move your fingers down and toward the center a little you may find that this ligament is also sore. Pain in a rectangular area approximately 3cm horizontal by 10cm vertical as marked on the diagram has been shown to indicate sacroiliac problems.[1,2]

Look at your body diagram. If you circled areas of bony tenderness *on the same side you are having your symptoms, then start with exercises #1 and #2* in order to balance out the muscles in your pelvis. When these areas of bony tenderness improve (usually within a few days), then progress to exercises #3 and #4. If you have similar tenderness on *both sides, or no tenderness* in these areas, skip exercise #1 and *begin your program with exercises #2, #3 and #4.* However, please continue reading the following information on breathing, which applies to everyone.

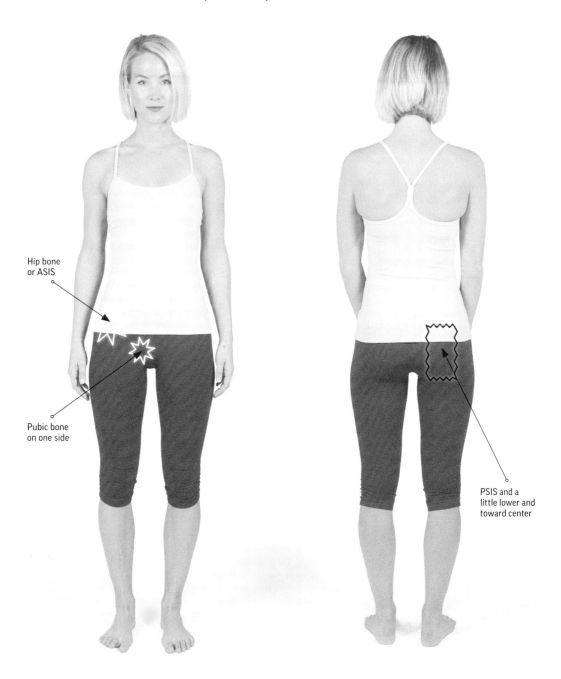

Figure 14.

Breathing

First, let's get the breathing right. While doing these exercises it is best to breathe using your diaphragm, the large breathing muscle located under your lungs. Figure 15 is a drawing of your lungs located beneath your rib cage.

There are small muscles between your ribs that contract and work with your diaphragm to help open up your rib cage so your lungs can expand with your breath. Some people have not used these muscles in a while, so if your rib cage does not move out to the sides when you are breathing deeply, you may need to work on this separately. This won't prevent these exercises from working for you, but good deep breathing is beneficial for many reasons. One of these reasons is to reduce stress or anxiety and pain. (We will talk about this more in **Step 2, deep core exercise #4.**)

Place your hands on the sides of your ribs (Figure 16). Take a deep breath in, thinking about moving your rib cage out into your hands (like opening up an umbrella), and let your belly muscles relax. Relaxing your belly will allow the diaphragm to contract and move down and increase your rib cage space from the bottom. Slowly exhale to at least the count of five. Try quieting your brain and relaxing all your muscles. For relaxing effects, do this eight to 10 times in a row.

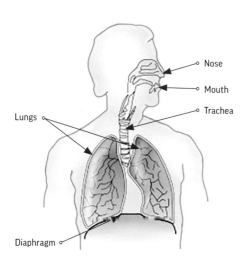

Figure 15. Lungs

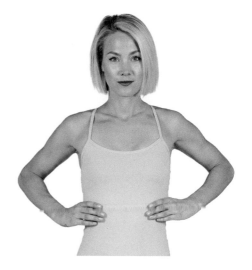

Figure 16.

Pelvic balancing exercise #1

This exercise is recommended to be performed as described below (with left knee up and lifting right buttock off the ground) **no matter what side the pain is on, right or left**, unless directed by a therapist. This is based on the predominate patterns seen in sacroiliac dysfunction.

Start by lying down on your back and bringing your left knee toward you. Place your left hand on your left knee and take a deep breath in (Figure 17). While slowly exhaling, push your left hand into your left knee with moderate pressure, and push down with your right foot (push more through the heel if you can), lifting your right buttock up a few inches (Figure 18). It will feel like one smooth movement done with the slow exhale. Then slowly lower with the inhale.

Perform one set of 10-15 repetitions. You may want to repeat another set later in the day if your "bony tenderness signs" return or worsen. As your muscles balance in your pelvis, you will no longer have these tender spots and will not need to perform this exercise. This exercise may be painful at first but this should improve by the time you are done with your first set. (It is OK to start with two to three sets of five repetitions if 10 feels too difficult.) Try not to push as hard or lift as high if you are having difficulty. It is not necessary to come off the floor with your buttock, just pushing down with your foot and thinking about lifting your buttock is a good starting place. If you are having trouble coordinating the breathing, just make sure you are not holding your breath, especially while pushing. This will make the exercise less effective or not effective at all.

Additional tip: Keep your right foot close to your buttock in this exercise to avoid getting hamstring (back of thigh) cramps. This encourages the buttocks (gluteus maximus) muscle to work more, and this muscle is often weak.

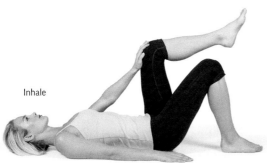

Figure 17.

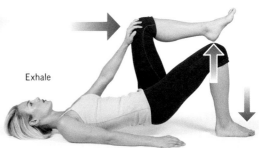

Figure 18.

Watch video: **OPTP.com/RiczoVideos**

Pelvic balancing exercise #2A

Start by lying down on your back. Take a deep breath in through your nose slowly and think about expanding your rib cage and relaxing your belly while moving your knees out to the side, moving heels toward each other (Figure 19). Then slowly exhale and move knees together and your toes together, gently squeezing your knees together (Figure 20).

(If it is painful moving your toes in or heels in then do not do this part for the first three to four days. Then try it again. Do what you can.)

Move in a range that's comfortable for you when moving your knees out and in, relaxing the rest of your body. Do not force. More is not better in this situation. It might be painful at first but will get better as you continue and focus on your breathing and relaxing.

Perform at least 30 repetitions. Stop if you need to at 10 or 15 repetitions, rest and then continue. Try to do three sets a day. This is to create relaxation and balance in these muscles throughout the day, and to help create a mindfulness of relaxation.

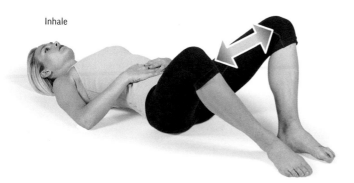

Figure 19.

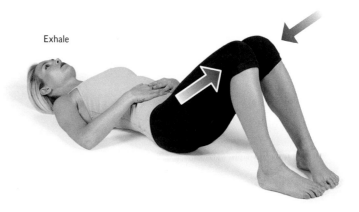

Figure 20.

Watch video: **OPTP.com/RiczoVideos**

Pelvic balancing exercise #2B

When exercise #2A becomes easy you can progress this exercise by adding a stretchy exercise band and pillow as in Figure 21. You will be pushing out on the band with the inhale (Figure 21) and squeezing on the pillow with the exhale (Figure 22). If this causes you pain, then reduce the effort and make sure you are just using your legs for the contraction, not tensing up the rest of your body. If it still causes you pain, then return to exercise #2A without the pillow and band. Perform two to three sets of 10 to 15 repetitions once a day. As you get stronger you can work toward two sets of 15 repetitions, then progress to one set of 30. Rest between sets for approximately 45 to 60 seconds.

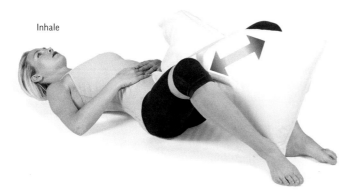

Figure 21.

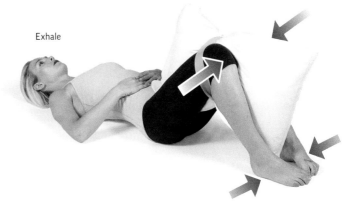

Figure 22.

Watch video: **OPTP.com/RiczoVideos**

Pelvic balancing exercise #2C

When you feel stronger, progress exercise #2B by adding a buttock lift as in Figure 23 and lowering as in Figure 24. The breathing, hip, and leg movement is the same as in #2A and #2B.

Perform three sets of 10 to 15 repetitions once a day. As you get stronger you can work toward two sets of 15 repetitions, then progress to one set of 30. Rest between sets for approximately 45 to 60 seconds.

Additional tip: You can do this exercise without the resistance band or pillow. This is a variation that will make this exercise less difficult.

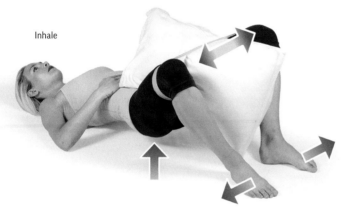

Figure 23.

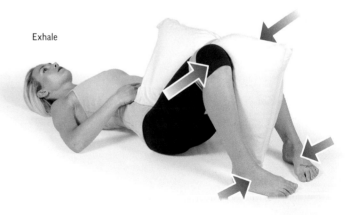

Figure 24.

Watch video: **OPTP.com/RiczoVideos**

Pelvic balancing exercise #3

Begin exercise #3 when your bony tenderness (as described on pg. 11, Figure 14) has lessened, and your right and left sides feel similar. (This tenderness should improve by performing exercises #1 and #2.) If this one-sided bony tenderness has not been an issue for you, you will skip exercise #1 and perform exercises #2 and #3.

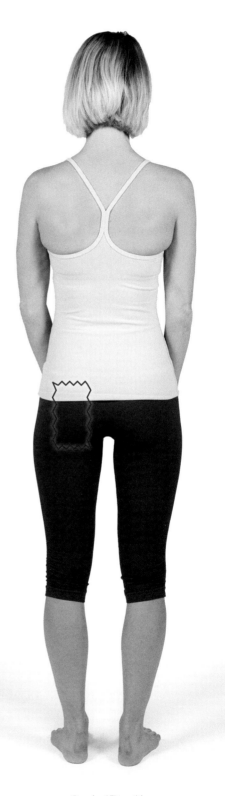

Sample of Figure 14.

Pelvic balancing exercise #3 continued

Sit tall on a firm chair without arms (bed is OK if chair not available). Start with your pain-free side. Bend that knee and tuck your foot in toward your opposite thigh in as comfortable position as possible. Use a stool to rest your foot in front of you if you cannot get your foot on the seat or bed.

Press down gently on your bent knee with the opposite hand and turn to that side as far as comfortably possible, thinking about turning from the waist. Breathe slowly and think about your rib cage moving out with each inward breath and your stomach muscles relaxing. Sit evenly on both sit bones (bones in your buttocks that you sit on), and hold this position for 10 seconds. Return to facing forward, keeping your leg in the same position.

Repeat this on the same side two more times for a total of three times. Then repeat this same exercise on your other side (painful side) for one set of three repetitions. You most likely will not be able to turn as far; that is OK. You may feel pulling; that is good as we want to stretch these tissues. Then repeat again on each side; one more set of three repetitions.

The second set on your painful side should feel better. Remember to sit tall. The key is to relax into the movement. Do not force any movement. Repeat two to three times a day as needed. You should feel better after this exercise. If you don't, check to see if:

- You are shifting off of your sit bones (stay even on sit bones)
- You are trying too hard as you are turning
- You are holding your breath (breathe!)
- You are going into sharp pain (do not turn so far)

If none of the above is happening, then this may not be the right exercise for you; do not continue to do this exercise.

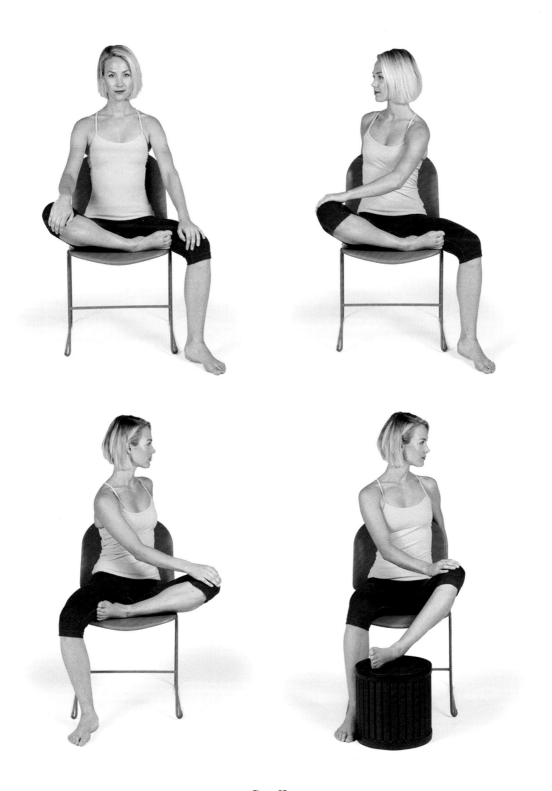

Figure 25.

Watch video: **OPTP.com/RiczoVideos**

Step 2. Activating your deep core muscles

Let's review a little research on how muscles work first. Activating your deep core is a powerful exercise for everyone. These muscles become weak as we age, have children, gain weight, have injuries, surgeries (especially abdominal or back), have physical jobs, episodes of back pain, high stress, or sedentary lives. They all work together rhythmically and without thought in the normal functioning person. We benefit by having good postural control of our spine, a responsive respiratory system, and bowel and bladder control.[3,4]

In addition, breath awareness and conscious relaxation is known to be a very powerful tool to lower pain. This is because deep breathing affects our neurological system, namely our sympathetic and parasympathetic nervous system.[5]

Deep breathing triggers our parasympathetic nervous system to calm down our sympathetic nervous system. The sympathetic nervous system is responsible for preparing us to respond to danger. This is known as the "fight or flight" response. The sympathetic nervous system is "on fire" when we are in fear, have anxiety, and/or have pain. It releases stress hormones, which continues the vicious cycle of chronic pain.[6] If we are "on fire" all the time this becomes very unhealthy for our bodies.

Being aware of our bodies and our present feelings and situation without judgment is also important for our well-being. This is called mindfulness. There is plenty of good information available about mindfulness, and I would encourage you to read more on this topic.[7]

Activating your deep core, exercise #4

This exercise engages the diaphragm, deep abdominals (transversus abdominus), deep back muscles (multifidi) and pelvic floor muscles. Lie on your back with knees straight or bent, hips lying on a wedge or pillow if your pelvic floor is very weak (Figure 26), or hips just on floor (Figure 27).

Take a deep breath in (remember, think about your rib cage opening up like an umbrella). If you place one hand on your upper chest and think about quieting the up and down movement of your chest, this may help you focus on opening up like an umbrella from the bottom of your ribs (Figure 27).

As you exhale through pursed lips (like blowing up a balloon or with a hissing noise), contract your pelvic floor muscles by thinking about stopping gas or the flow of urine (or both). You will feel a lifting up of your pelvic floor and a tightening, drawing in of your lower abdominals. You can place one hand on your lower abdominals (Figure 27) to encourage these muscles, your transverse abdominus muscles, to flatten. A good visual for getting these muscles to contract more is thinking about what you do when zipping up a pair of tight jeans.

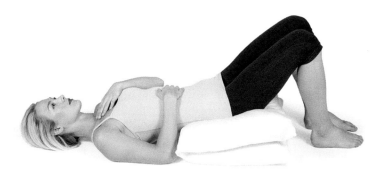

Figure 26.

Easy, relaxing breathing throughout this exercise. Hand placement near lower ribs to check if ribs are opening up like an umbrella. Use pillows under hips if pelvic floor muscles are weak so pelvis is inclined.

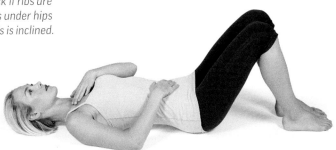

Figure 27.

Hand placement on lower abdomen to check if abdominals are flattening as you exhale (as if blowing up a balloon or with a hissing sound).

As you repeat this exercise, use the above imagery (umbrella, balloon/hissing, stopping urine/gas, zipping up zipper) to help you be more effective in getting these muscles to contract well. It will also help you to slow down your breath so you can contract longer. Exhaling slowly also automatically triggers the correct muscles.

If this exercise causes you pain, change your position so you can do it comfortably. You can do this exercise lying on your stomach with a pillow under your stomach, on your side, on hands and knees, and in sitting or standing. It is best to do this exercise in a variety of positions to challenge your muscles differently (because of gravity).

If your pelvic floor is painful when you contract, then focus on the relaxation part of the exercise and less on the contraction of the pelvic floor muscle (the stopping urine/gas portion). Make sure you relax your belly muscles when you are inhaling as that will help relax the pelvic floor muscles.

Perform sets of 8 to 10 repetitions three to four times a day to build up your strength and endurance in your deep core muscles. Be mindful of having good posture in whatever position you choose (lying, sitting, standing, hands and knees). Try to avoid having your rib cage tipped up or down. Think about the umbrella imagery and that the umbrella is open evenly. Tipping the umbrella up in front would look like standing in a military posture while tipping it down would look like standing slumped.

It is best to spread out the sets during the day to remind yourself of the power of the breath and to wake up these muscles in general. Being mindful of relaxing extra tension will bring in a side benefit of reducing stress.

This exercise will help strengthen your pelvic floor muscles. It is important to have normal functioning of our pelvic floor muscles as these muscles contribute to the control of our urine and bowels, provide organ support, and help sexual functioning. So when these muscles are not functioning properly we can have problems with urine or bowel control, prolapse of our bladders, uterus or rectum, and painful or not pleasurable intercourse.

Of course there may be other reasons you are experiencing these symptoms. A thorough evaluation by your gynecologist, uro-gynecologist, or certified pelvic floor physical therapist is a good place to begin for guidance and treatment. In the United States you do not need a referral to see a physical therapist; however, some larger hospital facilities and others still require a physician's referral.

You can "Find a PT" at the American Physical Therapy Association (APTA) website MoveForwardPT.com. You will search by your zip code initially but can specify specialty area in the drop down box. For a pelvic floor therapist, choose Women's Health. (This name may soon be changed to something related to Pelvic Health.)

When you improve your control with activating these muscles you can do this exercise without the pursed lips or hissing noise, and work on these muscles even when standing in line!

Step 3. Stretching your buttocks, hips and low back; achieving balance between the sides of your body

First some tips. There are many stretches that are great to do and will improve your flexibility. In this section there are common stretches that address important flexibility problems found in persons with sacroiliac issues. Here are important principles to keep in mind.

- Muscles stretch better when they are warm. So if you have just gotten out of bed, been sitting for a long time, or been outside in the cold it is best to warm up your muscles first. This can be done with a warm shower, dynamic stretching (as is often done before soccer or baseball, such as high stepping, walking lunges, walking squats), or just moving in general.

- Muscles respond better to slow stretching rather than fast movement to your end range. Moving fast brings in an automatic protective mechanism in the muscle that causes the muscle to contract. This is to protect the joint from injury. So if the movement is done too quickly the muscle actually contracts or tightens instead of being stretched.

- Breathing into the stretch and relaxing the rest of your body will encourage relaxation in the muscle you are trying to stretch.

- You do not need to stretch muscles that are already lengthened. For example, many people who have over-lengthened hamstrings still like to stretch them, but they can already bring their nose to their knee. These muscles most likely need to be strengthened instead.

- Both sides of your body, meaning the right side and the left side, should feel about the same in flexibility and strength. Be aware of any one-sided tightness as you stretch and concentrate more on the tight side. If your non-painful side does not feel tight, you can shorten the time you are holding and even skip the repetition. The recommendation for stretching is to perform two sets, holding for 30 seconds on each side, once per day.

- It would be beneficial to perform the exercises that address your extra tight muscles a few additional times during the day. Modifications that are in sitting and standing are usually easier to perform during the day and can be effective.

Remember the principles in this bulleted list!

Some of these stretches can be enhanced with the OPTP® Stretch Out Strap®, a nylon woven (non-elastic) strap for improving flexibility and range of motion. The Stretch Out Strap safely delivers all the benefits of assisted stretching without the need for a partner and is available at OPTP.com

Knee to chest stretch

You can do this stretch with the straight leg bent if it is more comfortable. Keeping your leg straight also works on stretching your hip flexor muscle, which we will address in this section. You may find it more comfortable to use a strap, towel, or sheet to assist with this stretch as shown in the variations. Perform two sets, holding for 30 seconds on each side, once per day. Breathe into the stretch.

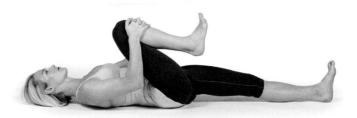

Figure 28.
Knee to chest stretch. Stretches out low back and hip muscles.

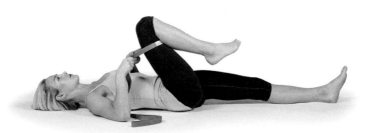

Figure 29.
Knee to chest variation with Stretch Out Strap.

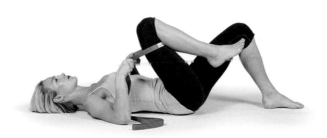

Figure 30.
Knee to chest variation with Stretch Out Strap and bent knee.

Piriformis stretch

Keep your shoulders flat as you bring your leg across your body. Use a towel or strap around your thigh if you have difficulty holding your leg. Use the sitting variation (Figure 33) to get more repetitions in during your day. Perform two sets, holding for 30 seconds on each side, once per day. Breathe into the stretch.

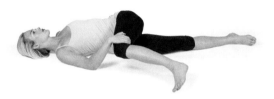

Figure 31.
Crossover piriformis stretch.
Stretches out the small hip rotators and low back muscles.

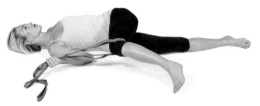

Figure 32.
Crossover piriformis stretch variation.

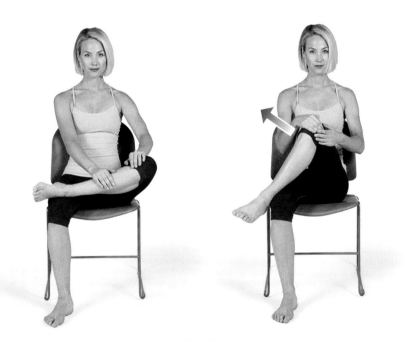

Figure 33.
Sitting crossover piriformis stretch variation. Remember to use this variation if your muscles are tight.

Figure of 4 stretch (small hip rotator muscles including the piriformis)

The piriformis muscle actually needs to be stretched in two different positions, one with your knee in a direction away from your body (Figure 34) and the other with your knee crossing your body as in the previous exercise.

You can begin with Figure 34 and gently push down on the bent knee, holding for 30 seconds, and then repeat again. If this feels difficult you can move your foot that is on the ground further away from your buttock.

When this becomes less of a stretch, advance to bringing your thigh toward you as in Figure 35. Use a strap, towel, or sheet if this feels more comfortable (Figure 36). Perform two sets, holding for 30 seconds on each side, once per day. Breathe into the stretch.

You can also perform this stretch in sitting as in Figure 37. As these muscles become more flexible you can even lean forward as in the Figure 37 sitting variation.

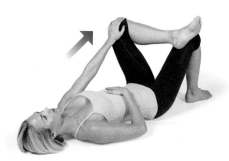

Figure 34.
Figure of 4 stretch, stretches small hip rotator.

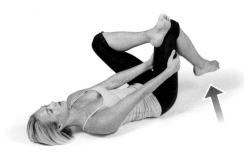

Figure 35.
Figure of 4 stretch variation, advanced.

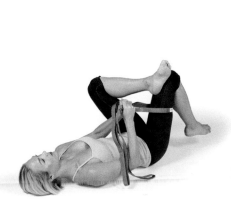

Figure 36.
Figure of 4 stretch variation with Stretch Out Strap.

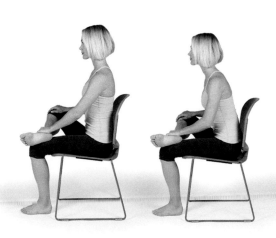

Figure 37.
Figure of 4 stretch sitting variation.

Hamstring/calf stretch (muscle in back of thigh/calf)

The hamstrings attach to your pelvis, and when they are tight they pull on your pelvis. The stretch position in Figure 38 is a good stretch to start with because your back is supported by the floor and it also stretches your calf if you have the strap around the bottom of your foot.

Another common way to stretch your hamstrings is in sitting (Figure 39). You need to keep your back straight and bend at the hips to feel the stretch in your hamstrings, and pull your toes toward you to feel the stretch in your calf.

You can also add a towel, sheet, or strap to this variation (Figure 40). Perform two sets, holding for 30 seconds on each side, once per day. Breathe into the stretch.

The inverted V is a more advanced and dynamic stretch that also works your upper body (Figure 41). It is an excellent progression when you are able to tolerate it. You may recognize this as a popular yoga position when the knees are straight; downward dog. You can shift weight from leg to leg like you are stepping to make it a dynamic stretch. Hold each stretch for two to three seconds, alternating back and forth for a total of approximately 30 seconds. Rest approximately 45-60 seconds. Repeat.

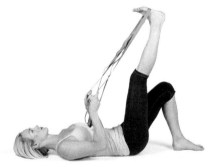

Figure 38.
Hamstring stretch with Stretch Out Strap.

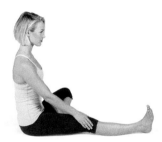

Figure 39.
Hamstring stretch sitting variation.

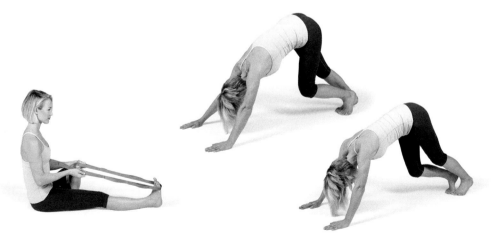

Figure 40.
Hamstring/calf stretch sitting variation with Stretch Out Strap.

Figure 41.
Hamstring/calf stretch variation inverted V.

Hip flexor stretch (muscle flexes the hip, stretch felt in groin/thigh)

The hip flexor muscles attach the spine and pelvis to your leg (femur) and work to flex your hip. They are often tight due to sitting and poor posture. In the first stretch in half kneeling (Figure 42) you can hold onto a chair or other surface for balance at first. If needed you can put a small towel under the knee for cushion. Remember to keep your trunk straight. It is also important to tighten your abdominals, particularly the transversus abdominus muscle (the zipping up a tight pair of jeans muscle) as well as tightening the buttock. This helps to target the hip flexor muscle.

If the hip flexor muscle is tight you will feel the stretch in Figure 42. If you do not feel the stretch, lean slowly forward until you do as in Figure 43. Progress to work on balance without holding on, even switching from side to side without holding on for support. Perform two sets, holding for 30 seconds on each side, once per day. Breathe into the stretch.

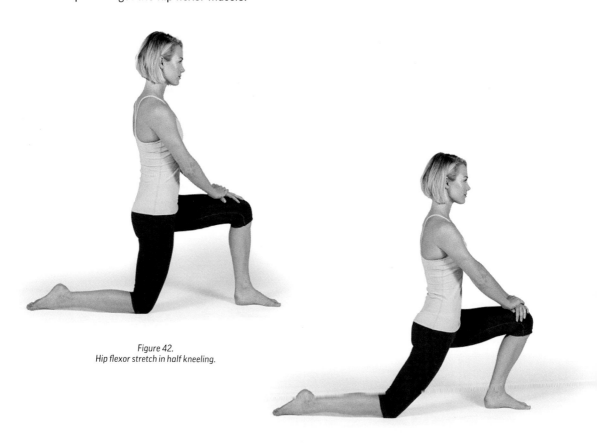

Figure 42.
Hip flexor stretch in half kneeling.

Figure 43.
Hip flexor stretch in half kneeling with lean variation.

Calf/hip flexor stretch in standing position

The calf muscles located in the back of our legs are often tight due to lack of stretching and shoe wear (high heels). When they are tight the dynamics of our walking and stressors on our body increase. The standing calf stretch (Figure 44) is one of the common calf stretches. This stretch, when you contract your stomach muscles (transversus abdominus) and even your buttock muscle on the leg that is behind you, will also stretch your hip flexor on that side. Perform two sets, holding for 30 seconds on each side, once per day. Breathe into the stretch.

You can perform this stretch in standing using a chair as in Figure 45. This will also give you a good stretch in your calf muscles. Progress to adding the arm reach as in the third picture. If tighter on one side, then concentrate on that side until both feel similar. Perform two sets, holding for 30 seconds on each side, once per day. Breathe into the stretch.

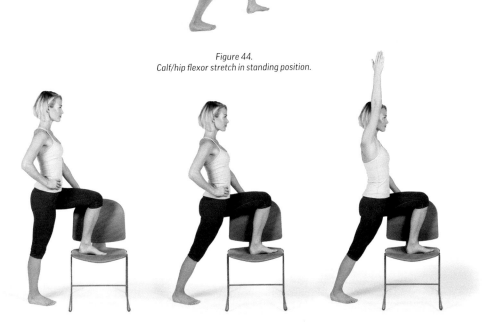

Figure 44.
Calf/hip flexor stretch in standing position.

Figure 45.
Calf/hip flexor stretch standing with chair variation.

Groin stretch (muscles on the inside of upper thigh)

These muscles attach to your pelvis and your leg (femur) and also affect the dynamics of your pelvis. Sit tall during this stretch (you can sit with your back to a wall as in Figure 47) and notice if one side is tighter than the other in your groin. You can apply a gentle pressure with your forearms to get a better stretch if this is comfortable (not painful). Perform two sets, holding for 30 seconds on each side, once per day. Breathe into the stretch.

Progress to the standing inner groin stretch (Figure 48). This involves balance and also works on strengthening of your legs and core as you maintain an upright trunk.

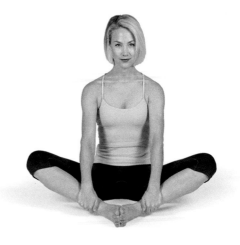

Figure 46.
Groin stretch addresses your inner thigh muscles.

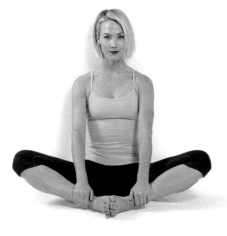

Figure 47.
Groin stretch variation using the wall for support.

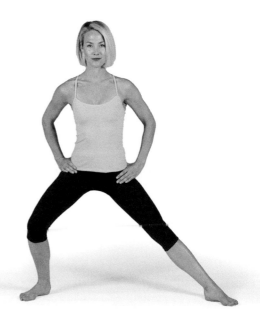

Figure 48.
Groin stretch standing variation; more advanced as it works on your leg strength, core, balance, and posture.

Step 4. Begin a walking program

If you are already walking for exercise, good for you! Walking has been shown to be one of the best exercises for fitness, and dog owners who walk their dogs have been shown to be more physically fit.[8,9] Of course, you do not need a dog to go for a nice healthy walk every day. Here are some tips:

- Dress appropriately, including good shoes, for indoor walking also.

- Stand tall with rib cage not tipped up or down (no military or slouched posture but a level open umbrella!).

- Be aware of your breath. No breath holding!

- Stay hydrated. Take water with you, especially in warm weather.

- Do not go out in the extreme weather conditions or if you are feeling ill.

- Use good judgement at all times.

- Start at a reasonable distance for you, even if it is a five-minute walk. Take a cane or walking aid if you need it.

- Take a friend to make it more fun.

- Mall or treadmill walking are great! There are many walking groups in existence. Start with your local rec center or Y to help you find a group, if you are interested.

- If you are starting with a short walk, think about going out once in the morning, and then again in the afternoon or evening. This will give your body enough time to rest in between and will allow you to progress at a faster pace.

- You should not be walking so fast that you cannot talk on the phone or to a friend. This is called the "talk test."

- When you are trying to improve your speed, take shorter, faster steps instead of trying to take longer steps.

- Make an exercise calendar and record your time and sessions on each day.

- You can make extra copies of the Exercise and Stretching Planner at the back of this book to start. A fitness tracker (for example a Fitbit, Garmin, Apple watch) can also help with tracking exercise, walking and movement during the day.

- Set goals for yourself. Aim to increase three to five minutes from week to week. For example, if you walked for 15 minutes once a day for five days last week, see if you can do 20 minutes the following week. There are many other ways to progress time or distance, this is just a simplified plan.

- Your minutes walked may be different than the example above, but the idea is that you progress slowly. You should feel better at the end of each walk. If not, you may have gone too far or pushed yourself too much. That is fine, just make adjustments in your program by reducing the time walked, terrain (hills vs. flat), etc., or time of day (more energy first thing in the morning or midday).

Step 5. Progress to other physical activities that you enjoy, make healthy choices

You will be more likely to continue being active if you choose activities you enjoy, whether they be alone or with a friend. Consider activities such as hiking, biking, swimming, and more aggressive strengthening such as weightlifting and higher level core exercises.

Choose **wellness** and let that be a guiding principle when you are making decisions. It makes decisions much easier! If we don't choose wellness in our life by default we will be influenced by today's marketing, etc., which will tend to pull us in the other direction.

Everyone will progress through these steps of the Pelvic Girdle Musculoskeletal Method[SM] at their own pace. This will be influenced by their prior fitness level, age, weight, other orthopedic or neurologic conditions, motivation, emotional support, etc. It is important to view exercise not only as a means to "get rid of pain" but more so as a vehicle for general fitness, health and well-being.

Steps 1 through 3 are designed to assess and address the "balance of muscle strength and flexibility" in your body. This includes not only voluntary muscles of the legs and back but the involuntary muscles that are responsible for your breathing and deep core mechanisms.

Steps 4 and 5 are to help you transition to "choosing wellness" by making daily choices based on fitness and how it affects your quality of life. Healthy eating is a huge part of this wellness approach as food is the "fuel" we put into the "car." There is plenty written on healthy eating, and your doctor can direct you to a dietitian or nutritionist for professional help. If you are looking on the internet for advice, a good rule of thumb is to stick with ".org" or ".gov" website endings to avoid fake or unproven information.

One diet approach to look at is The DASH diet, originally designed for high blood pressure. It is also in line with dietary recommendations to prevent osteoporosis, cancer, heart disease, stroke, and diabetes. DASH stands for Dietary Approaches to Stop Hypertension and is a highly recommended diet.[10]

These steps are guidelines. Your physical therapist is well educated to help you through them. Another great resource of reliable health information is the consumer education site of the American Physical Therapy Association; **MoveForwardpt.com**

Good luck on your journey!

References

1. Fortin JD, Vilensky JA, Merkel GM. Can the Sacroiliac Joint Cause Sciatica? *Pain Physician*. 2003;(6):269-271.

2. Vleeming A, Pool-Goudzwaard AL, Hammudoghlu D, Stoeckart R, Snijders CJ, Mens JM. The function of the long dorsal sacroiliac ligament: its implication for understanding low back pain. *Spine*. 1996;21(5):556-562.

3. Hodges PW, Gandevia SC. Activation of the human diaphragm during a repetitive postural task. *J Physiol*. 2000;522(Pt 1):165-175. doi:10.1111/j.1469-7793.2000.t01-1-00165.xm.

4. Lee, DG. *The Pelvic Girdle: An Integration of Clinical Expertise and Research*. 4th ed. Churchill Livingstone; 2011.

5. Busch V, Magerl W, Kern U, Haas J, Hajak G, Eichhammer P. The Effect of Deep and Slow Breathing on Pain Perception, Autonomic Activity, and Mood Processing—An Experimental Study. *Pain Med*. 2012;13(2):215-228. doi:10.1111/j.1526-4637.2011.01243.x.

6. Publishing HH. Understanding the stress response. Harvard Health. https://www.health.harvard.edu/staying-healthy/understanding-the-stress-response. Published March 2011. Accessed September 20, 2017.

7. Mindfulness | Definition | Greater Good Magazine. https://greatergood.berkeley.edu/mindfulness/definition. Accessed September 20, 2017.

8. Cutt H, Giles-Corti B, Knuiman M, Burke V. Dog ownership, health and physical activity: a critical review of the literature. *Health Place*. 2007;13(1):261-272. doi:10.1016/j.healthplace.2006.01.003.

9. Christian HE, Westgarth C, Bauman A, et al. Dog ownership and physical activity: a review of the evidence. *J Phys Act Health*. 2013;10(5):750-759.

10. DASH diet: Healthy eating to lower your blood pressure. Mayo Clinic. http://www.mayoclinic.org/healthy-lifestyle/nutrition-and-healthy-eating/in-depth/dash-diet/art-20048456. Accessed September 15, 2017.

SECTION THREE

Other helpful information

Using a sacroiliac belt

A sacroiliac belt is designed to support the sacroiliac joint by providing compression to the joint. In a normal functioning person without sacroiliac pain, the muscles, ligaments, bony structure of the sacrum and ilium, the motor control (or patterns of muscles being used), and emotional awareness of the person combine together to provide this support.[1] Research supports the use of a sacroiliac belt during pregnancy in women who have sacroiliac pain.[2]

To determine if you would benefit from a sacroiliac belt, the best thing to do is to try it on. However, if it does not feel good, I would recommend checking to see if you have "bony tenderness signs" in your pelvis. Proceed through the exercises until these signs are mostly gone. At this point it would be appropriate to try a sacroiliac belt. It should feel good and supportive, not just like you have a tight belt on. If you don't have access to a belt, you can try wearing a regular, thicker belt around your hips over the sacral area to see if that provides some comfort. Do not put it on too tight.

There are several SI belts available on the market that can help relieve SI-related pain in the low back, hip, and pelvis, as well as referred sciatic pain in the leg. The Serola Sacroiliac Belt has been endorsed by the APTA Section on Women's Health. It is available on my website, RiczoHealthEducation.com. I also have a YouTube video from Riczo Health Education on how to put it on and some other tips.

The SI-LOC® is another good option, designed by the International Academy of Orthopedic Medicine, and is available at OPTP.com. Talk with your therapist and get a recommendation for which sacroiliac belt might be best for you. Your therapist can also help you ensure the proper fit during a consultation.

If the belt gives you some relief, I would recommend wearing it while exercising as well, and most of the day for two to three months. If rolling over in bed is very painful, it can be worn at night. As your muscles become stronger from exercising and you increase your activity level, you will find you won't need the belt any longer. At this point it will just feel like you are wearing a tight belt.

FAQs

1. **Should I use heat or ice for pain?**
   Generally, it is recommended to use ice to ease pain that results from inflammation and swelling. It works well for high levels of pain and causes a numbing effect while actually decreasing the inflammation. Heat is recommended after the inflammation resolves and helps with joint stiffness and relaxing tense muscles. You do not want to use heat with a new or acute injury or sudden flare-up of an old injury as it can increase inflammation and slow healing.[3] Apply ice to the area over a thin towel for approximately 10 minutes at a time, three to four times a day. Allow the tissues to come back to normal between applications. Apply heat for 15 to 20 minutes at a time, again allowing for time in between, applying three to four times a day. Be careful not to burn your skin or give yourself frostbite! If you can't see the area, use a mirror. I have seen damaged skin from overuse of ice and heat.

2. **I have been told I have a long leg. Should I wear a heel lift?**
   Often when muscles are tight on one side of your body it can feel or appear that one leg is longer than the other. Performing the "pelvic balancing exercises" in Section 2, Step 1 may very well take care of this feeling or appearance. If not, you have two choices. You can try a small heel lift (⅛ to ¼ inch) on the short side and see if it makes you feel better. Of course you have to continue wearing a shoe with a heel lift when you are inside your home to give this an honest trial. Some people use slippers or walk barefoot or with socks when at home. If you feel better with the heel lift you would need to continue wearing the heel lift in your shoe most of the time when you are on your feet. The second choice is to consult a physical therapist (preferably board certified in orthopedics), an orthopedic doctor, or podiatrist for an opinion and direction.

3. **My chiropractor has been giving me adjustments. I feel better for a while but have had these done for years. Should I keep going for these adjustments?**

   I would advise you to make a commitment to the program in this book without having other things influencing your symptoms. In this way you can determine what is making you feel better or worse, and if the exercises need to be modified. Remember, we are not moving bones or doing manipulation with this program, we are addressing muscle imbalances, weakness and strength, and, of course, addressing stress and the power of mindfulness.

4. **What exercises should I avoid?**

   While working through this program, I would recommend avoiding high impact exercises, such as jogging, running, high-impact aerobics, and those with fast-paced and quick turns such as soccer and basketball. Use of a sacroiliac belt would allow a quicker return to these activities as it would provide the sacroiliac joint more support. The best rule of thumb is to return at a gradual pace to determine your muscular endurance. For example, you may be able to jog for 10 minutes but start having pain at 12 minutes because the muscles are fatiguing. Some people just continue to push through the pain until they cannot bear it. I do not recommend this approach because it does not make physiological sense. A calendar to help you track your endurance would be helpful as described in Section 1.

5. **Can I take a vacation from exercise?**

   We all take "vacations" from exercise, either planned or unplanned. Your body will let you know if it is too long of a "vacation," either by a return of your symptoms, or by just not feeling as good as you did when you were exercising regularly. As long as you have made the overall commitment to choosing wellness for your life, you will return to regular exercise, hopefully sooner rather than later. The important thing to keep in mind is that you have not "failed" at keeping a regular program; do not continue beating yourself up about this. Just be mindful and return to an exercise program you enjoy. Keep this book handy if you should have your sacroiliac symptoms come back, and then return to the exercises in Section 2.

6. **Can I use a foam roller during this program?**

   Yes. A foam roller is very beneficial to address muscle tenderness and tightness. I would recommend, however, not using a roller if you have "bony tenderness signs." Work through the program in Section 2, Step 2 first until these signs resolve. Areas to target with the roller are the side and front of your thigh, buttocks, front of the hip, and low back. There is plenty of information on YouTube and in print for reference on how to use a foam roller. Visit **OPTP.com** for books such as *Foam Roller Techniques* and *PRO-ROLLER Massage Essentials*, along with many different sizes and densities of foam rollers.

7. **I have been having discomfort in my pelvic muscles. Is there anything I can do for this?**
Being mindful of your breath, overall body tension, and levels of stress can be very helpful. Often, these pelvic floor muscles tighten up because of stress and improper breathing patterns. As we inhale our diaphragm descends and abdominals relax. At this point there should be a coordinated relaxing of the pelvic floor muscles (automatically). As we exhale, the pelvic floor muscles should tighten and lift somewhat (we don't really feel this), the deep abdominals contract, and the diaphragm rises. This has been described as a pistoning motion.[4] When this pistoning action is lost through shallow breathing it can affect the pelvic floor.

Of course, there are other reasons the pelvic floor can be painful that are beyond the scope of this book. One tool that can be helpful in increasing awareness of these muscles so you can improve their function is the PFProp™, also available from OPTP. It is a foam cylinder that can be used for sitting exercises that awaken and activate pelvic floor muscles. It aids in promoting pelvic and core strength, healthful posture, balance, and flexibility. In addition to helping counteract the negative effects of prolonged sitting, it is also helpful for anyone with compromised pelvic floor strength. The PFProp includes exercise instruction, and more information is available on OPTP's website at **OPTP.com/PFProp.**

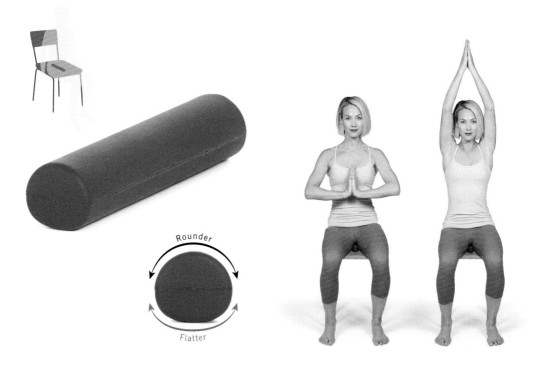

Exercise planner

Make eight copies of this page and use one page per week.   WEEK #..........

Exercise	Page #	Reps/sets/per day recommended	My reps/sets/per day	M	T	W	TH	F	SA	SU
Pelvic Balancing #1	13	10-15 reps 1 set 1 to 2x day								
#2a	14	30 reps 1 set 3x day								
#2b	15	10-15 reps 2-3 sets 1x day								
#2c	16	10-15 reps 3 sets 1x day								
#3	17	10 seconds hold x 3 each side, non-painful side first. 2 sets 2-3x day as needed								
#4 Deep Core	21	8-10 reps 3-4x day, lying on stomach, back, side, sitting, standing, hands and knees								
Walking	31	15 minutes per day, 5x week Increase each week	My Time:							

Stretching planner

Make eight copies of this page and use one page per week.   WEEK #..........

Stretches	Page #	Reps/sets/per day recommended	My reps/sets/per day	M	T	W	TH	F	SA	SU
Knee to chest	24	30 seconds each side 2 sets, 1x day								
Piriformis stretch	25	30 seconds each side 2 sets, 1x day								
Piriformis stretch, sitting	25	30 seconds each side 2 sets, 1x day								
Figure of 4 stretch, lying	26	30 seconds each side 2 sets, 1x day								
Figure of 4 stretch, lying, advanced	26	30 seconds each side 2 sets, 1x day								
Figure of 4 stretch, sitting	26	30 seconds each side 2 sets, 1x day								
Hamstring stretch, lying	27	30 seconds each side 2 sets, 1x day								
Hamstring stretch, sitting	27	30 seconds each side 2 sets, 1x day								
Hamstring stretch, inverted V	27	30 seconds each side 2 sets, 1x day								
Hip flexor stretch, ½ kneel	28	30 seconds each side 2 sets, 1x day								
Hip flexor stretch, ½ kneel with lean	28	30 seconds each side 2 sets, 1x day								
Calf/Hip flexor stretch, standing	29	30 seconds each side 2 sets, 1x day								
Calf/Hip flexor stretch, standing using chair	29	30 seconds each side 2 sets, 1x day								
Groin stretch, sitting	30	30 seconds each side 2 sets, 1x day								
Groin stretch, standing	30	30 seconds each side 2 sets, 1x day								

Goals

Use this page to write a weekly goal for yourself that is meaningful. Make it something realistic that you need to work on, that would make you happy, or would decrease your stress. For example, "I will be mindful of my breathing three times a day," "I will take a 10-minute walk in the park," or "I will decrease my social media usage (stress reducer!)."

Keep a log of your goals here and look back on them to see how you are doing. You may want to write your weekly goal out on paper and leave it several places that you will see during the day so you don't forget.

Week #1 Goal:..
....
....

Week #2 Goal:..
....
....

Week #3 Goal:..
....
....

Week #4 Goal:..
....
....

Week #5 Goal:..
....
....

Week #6 Goal:..
....
....

Week #7 Goal:..
....
....

Week #8 Goal:..
....
....